CANCER

Seven Signs and Symptoms of Cancer that you must know,"

William D. Jordan,

TABLE OF CONTENT

WHAT CONSTITUTES CANCER
HOW DOES MALIGNANCY START?
WHEN CANCER GETS WIDER
VARIETY OF CANCER
UNEXPECTED LOSS OF WEIGHT
THE VALUE OF QUICK EVALUATION
PHARYNGEAL (THROAT) CANCER:

INTRODUCTION

How to Interpret the Warning Signs

Health is the most valuable thread in the fabric of our life. It permeates our encounters and shapes the story of our travels. But in the middle of our bodies' complexity, there are whispers—subtle cues that demand our attention. These are the cues that cause us to stop, think, and look for solutions.

Welcome to "7 Signs and Symptoms of Cancer," a comprehensive look at the subtleties of health. Within these pages, we decipher the mystery of body language, shedding light on the indicators that, when deciphered, might serve as our partners in the pursuit of timely identification and remediation.

WHY THIS IS IMPORTANT

With its quiet strides and elaborate masks, Cancer often makes itself known via minute adjustments. We arm ourselves with information as we examine the seven signs and symptoms; this armor enables us to identify, address, and, most importantly, promote a proactive attitude toward our health.

AWAITING YOU:

A Pathway to Conscience:

Every chapter acts as a guide to help you navigate the maze of possible signs. We interpret the body's signals so you may be equipped to see the small clues that point to the possibility of cancer.
True Tales, True Effects:

You will come across examples of resilience and success along the way—people who tackled these warning flags head-on and came out stronger. Their experiences provide light on the way, demonstrating to us that awareness is a source of power rather than just a tool.

Enabling You to Take Action:

The basis for empowerment is knowledge. We discuss each symptom and indication while offering advice, tools, and doable actions to promote proactive involvement with your health and wellbeing.

The Appeal for Knowledge:

This ebook is a light in a world where knowledge is everywhere but often hard to find. It provides clarity among the chaos. It asks you to become aware of your body's signals, pay attention to it, and tune in.

Are you prepared to go out on this awareness-raising journey? Accept these pages as a manual, a wellspring of wisdom, and an exhortation to action. Because information is not just power when it comes to our health, but also a lifeline—a thread that binds us to a future of well-informed decision-making and wellbeing.

Flip the page and start your adventure.

Recall that awareness involves both knowing and reacting. Let's work together to interpret the symptoms and indicators, enabling ourselves and the people we love to work toward a healthier, better-informed future.

WHAT CONSTITUTES CANCER

An illness known as cancer occurs when some body cells proliferate out of control and invade other bodily regions.

With billions of cells making up the human body, cancer may begin practically anywhere. Human cells typically divide to create new cells as needed by the body by growing and multiplying. New cells replace old ones when they die as a result of aging or injury.

This controlled mechanism may sometimes malfunction, causing damaged or aberrant cells to proliferate and expand when they shouldn't. Tumors are lumps of tissue that may be formed by these cells. Cancerous or benign tumors may both occur.

Malignant tumors may metastasize, or spread into, neighboring tissues, and can even generate new tumors by traveling to far-off regions of the body. Malignant tumors is another term for cancerous tumors. Blood malignancies, including leukemias, often do not develop into solid tumors, but many cancers do.

Benign tumors do not penetrate or spread to neighboring tissues. Benign tumors seldom come back after removal, while malignant ones sometimes do. However, benign tumors may sometimes grow to be rather enormous. Some, like benign brain tumors, are potentially fatal or produce severe symptoms.

Characteristics of Normal Cells and Cancer Cells
a female information professional in the CIS.

Have inquiries? For answers, get in touch with a cancer information specialist.

Normal cells and cancer cells are not the same in many aspects. As an example, cancer cells

expand without receiving instructions to do so. Only in response to these cues can normal cells proliferate.
Disregard signals that ordinarily instruct cells to cease proliferating or to undergo programmed cell death, sometimes referred to as apoptosis.

infiltrate surrounding regions before spreading to other bodily parts. Most normal cells do not travel throughout the body; instead, they cease growing when they come into contact with other normal cells.
direct vascular growth in the direction of malignancies. These blood veins remove

waste materials from tumors and provide oxygen and nutrition to the tumors.

try to evade the immune system. Damaged or aberrant cells are often eliminated by the immune system.

elude the immune system and allow cancer cells to proliferate and survive. As an example, some cancer cells persuade immune cells to defend the tumor rather than to fight it.

acquire a variety of chromosomal modifications, including chromosome duplications and deletions. Some cancer cells contain twice as many chromosomes as healthy ones.

vary from regular cells in the kind of nutrition they need. Furthermore, unlike the majority of normal cells, certain cancer cells use nutrients in a different method to produce energy. This promotes the faster growth of cancer cells.

Cancer cells often depend on these aberrant activities so much that they are unable to function normally without them. Because of this, scientists have created treatments that specifically target the aberrant characteristics of cancer cells. Certain cancer treatments, for instance, stop blood vessels from expanding toward tumors, thereby depriving the tumor of vital nutrition.

HOW DOES MALIGNANCY START?

Certain alterations to genes, the fundamental building blocks of heredity, result in cancer. Chromosomes are lengthy strands of closely packed DNA that contain all of the genes.

Cancer is a hereditary illness, meaning that alterations to the genes that regulate our cells' growth and division are what cause cancer.

Cancer-causing genetic alterations may occur because:

of mistakes brought upon by cell division. of DNA deterioration brought on by toxic environmental elements like solar radiation and tobacco smoke's compounds.

Our parents passed them on to us.

Normally, damaged DNA cells are eliminated by the body before they become malignant. However, as we age, the body's capacity to do so decreases. This contributes to the increased risk of cancer in later life.

Everybody's cancer is caused by a different mix of genetic alterations. There will be further alterations as the cancer spreads. Different cells within the same tumor may have distinct genetic alterations.

The Basics of Cancer

Gene Types Involved in Cancer

Proto-oncogenes, tumor suppressor genes, and DNA repair genes are the three primary gene categories that are often impacted by the genetic alterations that lead to cancer. These alterations are sometimes referred to as cancer "drivers."

Proto-oncogenes play a role in the proper division and development of cells. On the other hand, these genes may become cancer-causing genes (also known as oncogenes), enabling cells to proliferate and survive when they shouldn't by changing in certain ways or becoming more active than usual.

Additionally, tumor suppressor genes regulate the division and development of cells. Certain tumor suppressor gene mutations may cause uncontrollably dividing cells.

Genes that repair damaged DNA are known as DNA repair genes. Mutations in these genes often lead to further mutations in other genes and chromosomal abnormalities such as duplications and deletions of chromosomal segments in the cells. When combined, these alterations have the potential to make the cells malignant.

Scientists have discovered that specific mutations are often present in a variety of cancer forms, as they continue to understand more about the molecular alterations that cause cancer. These days, a wide range of cancer therapies are available that focus on the gene abnormalities that cause cancer. Anybody with cancer who has the targeted mutation may utilize some of these therapies, regardless of the disease's initial growth site.

WHEN CANCER GETS WIDER

Cancer cells spread to other areas of the body and create new tumors there when they undergo metastasis.

Metastatic cancer is a kind of cancer that has spread to various parts of the body from its original site. Metastasis is the process by which cancer cells move to different areas of the body.

The initial, or primary, cancer and metastatic cancer have the same name and kind of cancer cells. For instance, breast cancer that spreads to the lung and develops into a tumor is called metastatic breast cancer, not lung cancer.

Metastatic cancer cells often have the same appearance as the initial cancer cells under a microscope. Furthermore, some molecular characteristics, such as the presence of certain chromosomal alterations, are often shared by the original cancer cell and metastatic cancer cells.

Treatment may, in some circumstances, help patients with metastatic cancer survive longer. In other instances, stopping the disease's spread or reducing its symptoms are the main objectives of therapy for metastatic cancer. The majority of cancer deaths are due to metastatic illness, and metastatic tumors may seriously impair a person's ability to operate.

CHANGES IN TISSUE THAT ARE NOT CANCER

Not every alteration in the tissues of the body is cancerous. However, if some tissue alterations are left untreated, they may progress to cancer. These are a few instances of tissue alterations that are not cancer but are sometimes under observation in case they develop into cancer:

When cells in a tissue proliferate more quickly than they should, an accumulation of additional cells is known as hyperplasia. Under a microscope, the tissue's organization and individual cells seem normal. Numerous causes or circumstances, including prolonged inflammation, may lead to hyperplasia.

Compared to hyperplasia, dysplasia is a more advanced disorder. An accumulation of extra cells is another feature of dysplasia. However, there are alterations in the tissue's organization and aberrant cell appearance. Generally speaking, cancer is more likely to develop in tissues and cells that seem aberrant. While certain forms of dysplasia need treatment or monitoring, others do not. A dysplastic nevus, a kind of aberrant mole that develops on the skin, is an example of dysplasia. Melanoma may develop from a dysplastic nevus, however, most do not.

The disease known as carcinoma in situ is considerably further advanced. Despite being referred to as stage 0 cancer sometimes, it is not cancer since the aberrant cells do not penetrate neighboring tissue in the same manner that cancer cells do. However, carcinomas in situ are routinely treated since some of them have the potential to develop into cancer.

Cancer cells may develop from normal cells. The aberrant alterations known as hyperplasia and dysplasia occur in cells before cancer cells develop in bodily tissues. An organ or tissue with hyperplasia has more cells that, when seen under a microscope, seem normal. Under a microscope, the cells in dysplasia seem aberrant, but they are not cancerous. Dysplasia and hyperplasia have the potential to develop into cancer.

VARIETY OF CANCER

Cancer comes in more than a hundred varieties. The organs or tissues where tumors originate are often used to designate different types of cancer. For instance, brain cancer begins in the brain, but lung cancer begins in the lung. Cancers may also be classified according to the kind of cell that gave rise to them, such as squamous or epithelial cells.

You may use our A to Z List of Cancers or the NCI website to search for information on certain cancer types depending on where the cancer is located in the body. Additionally, we have data about malignancies in children, adolescents, and young adults.

The following are some forms of malignancies that start in certain cell types:

CANCEROUS

The most frequent kind of cancer is carcinoma. Epithelial cells, which coat the body's exterior and interior surfaces, are responsible for their formation. There are several varieties of epithelial cells, which, when examined under a microscope, often resemble columns.

Specific designations are given to cancers that originate in distinct kinds of epithelial cells:

Adenocarcinoma is a kind of cancer that develops in mucous-producing epithelial cells. Sometimes, tissues containing this kind of epithelial cell are referred to as glandular tissues. Adenocarcinomas account for the majority of malignancies of the breast, colon, and prostate.

The bottom, or basal (base) layer of the epidermis, or a person's outermost layer of skin, is where basal cell carcinoma starts.

Squamous cells are epithelial cells that are located immediately below the skin's outer layer. Squamous cell carcinoma is a kind of cancer that develops in these cells. Numerous other organs, such as the stomach, intestines, lungs, bladder, and kidneys, are also lined by squamous cells. Squamous cells under a microscope have a flat appearance similar to fish scales. Epidermoid carcinomas are another name for squamous cell carcinomas.

A kind of epithelial tissue known as transitional epithelium, or urothelium, is where transitional cell carcinoma originates. This tissue is present in the linings of the bladder, ureters, kidneys (renal pelvis), and a few other organs. It is composed of many layers of epithelial cells that can change size. Transitional cell carcinomas may occur in some kidney, ureter, and bladder malignancies.

SARCOMA-LIKE

Muscles, tendons, fat, blood arteries, lymph vessels, nerves, and the tissue around joints are among the soft tissues of the body where soft tissue sarcoma may develop.

Cancers known as sarcomas may develop in the soft tissues of the bone, such as the muscles, fat, blood, and lymph arteries, as well as fibrous tissue (such as ligaments and tendons).

The most frequent cancer of the bone is osteosarcoma. Lipopolysarcoma, Kaposi sarcoma, liposarcoma, malignant fibrous histiocytoma, and dermatofibrosarcoma protuberans are the most prevalent forms of soft tissue sarcoma.

TERRORISM

Leukemias are cancers that start in the bone marrow's blood-forming tissue. Solid tumors are not formed by these cancers. Rather, a substantial number of aberrant white blood cells—leukemia cells and leukemic blast cells—accumulate in the bone marrow and circulation, displacing healthy blood cells. The body may find it more difficult to fight infections, regulate bleeding, and provide oxygen to its tissues if there is a low concentration of regular blood cells.

Leukemia comes in four basic forms, which are categorized according to the kind of blood cell the cancer begins in (lymphoblastic or myeloid) and the rate at which the illness progresses (acute or chronic). Leukemia grows more slowly in chronic types and more swiftly in acute variants.

LEUKEMIA

Cancer that starts in lymphocytes is known as lymphoblasts (T cells or B cells). These arc immune system-fighting white blood cells that combat illness. Abnormal lymphocytes accumulate in lymph nodes, lymph arteries, and other bodily organs in lymphoma.

Two primary forms of lymphoma exist:

Hodgkin lymphoma: Individuals with this illness have Reed-Sternberg cells, which are aberrant lymphocytes. Usually, B cells give rise to these cells.

Non-Hodgkin lymphoma is a broad category of malignancies that originate in the lymph nodes. B cells or T cells may give rise to malignancies, which can develop swiftly or slowly.

NUMEROUS MYELOMAS

Another kind of immune cell called a plasma cell is the source of multiple myeloma. Myeloma cells, which are aberrant plasma cells, accumulate in the bone marrow and develop into tumors in bones throughout the body. Kahler disease and plasma cell myeloma are other names for multiple myeloma.

For further information, see our article on different plasma cell neoplasms, including multiple myeloma.

ROSANOMA

Cancer that starts in cells that develop into melanocytes, which are specialized cells that produce melanin, the pigment responsible for the color of skin, is known as melanoma. Although melanomas most often occur on the skin, they may also develop in other pigmented tissues, such as the eye.

Spinal cord and brain tumors

Tumors of the brain and spinal cord may be of several kinds. The cellular type in which these tumors originated and the location of the tumor's initial formation inside the central nervous system is the basis for their names. For instance, astrocytes, which are star-shaped brain cells that support the health of nerve cells, are the starting point of an astrocytic tumor. Benign brain tumors (not cancerous) and malignant brain tumors (cancer).

For further information, see our article on malignancies of the brain and spinal cord.

OTHER TUMOR TYPES

Germ Cell Growths

One kind of tumor that starts in the cells that produce sperm or eggs is called a germ cell tumor. These tumors may be benign or malignant, and they can appear almost anywhere in the body.

A list of germ cell tumors with links to more information may be found on our page on malignancies by body region or system.

TUMORS NEUROENDOCRINE

Cells that release hormones into the blood in response to a signal from the neurological system give rise to neuroendocrine tumors. These tumors may produce a wide range of symptoms due to their potential to produce hormones in larger quantities than usual. Benign or malignant neuroendocrine tumors are both possible.

CARCINOID GROWTHS

Neuroendocrine tumors include carcinoid tumors. These are slow-growing tumors that are often detected in the small intestine and rectum of the gastrointestinal tract.

Carcinoid tumors may produce chemicals like prostaglandins or serotonin, which can lead to the development of carcinoid syndrome. They can also move to the liver or other parts of the body.

Seven Indicators of Cancer

- Unexpected Loss of Weight
- Tiredness
- Alterations in the Skin
- Continued Pain
- Modifications to Bladder or Bowel Habits
- Having Trouble Swallowing
- Chronic Cough or Hoarse Voice

UNEXPECTED LOSS OF WEIGHT

Unexpected weight loss may be a worrying sign that needs to be checked out, especially if it doesn't happen as a result of conscious dietary or activity modifications. Even while many people want to lose weight, inadvertently dropping a few pounds might be a sign of an underlying medical condition, such as cancer.

To further emphasize the relevance of inexplicable weight loss as a possible cancer indicator, consider the following:

Inadvertent Character:
One major area of worry is losing weight without making a deliberate attempt to do so. Without making any adjustments to their diet or exercise regimen, a person may experience a noticeable weight

reduction, which might be an indication of an underlying medical condition.

Metabolic Alterations:

The metabolism of the body may be impacted by cancer, which can cause fat and muscle tissue to break down quickly. This may lead to weight loss that is out of proportion to the person's caloric intake and degree of physical activity.

Cancer of the Digestive System:

Intestinal, pancreatic, and colorectal cancers are examples of digestive system tumors that may impede the body's absorption of nutrients. This malabsorption can cause weight loss even in cases when the individual is eating a typical diet.

A rise in energy consumption:

Weight loss may result from some tumors because they raise the body's energy consumption. Certain blood malignancies and hyperthyroidism are two examples of tumors that may exhibit this increased metabolic activity.

Diminished Appetite:

An appetite loss may be caused by cancer-related conditions, such as tumors or adverse effects from therapy. Over time, this decreased appetite may help with weight reduction.

The Cachexia

Cachexia is a disorder that may sometimes result from cancer and is marked by extreme weight loss, weakness, and muscular atrophy. Cachexia may have a serious negative effect on a person's general health and is often seen in the late stages of cancer.

THE VALUE OF QUICK EVALUATION

Even while losing weight on its own does not indicate that cancer is present, it is a sign that should not be disregarded. To determine the underlying reason, a healthcare professional's timely assessment is essential. Thyroid conditions, diabetes, or recurrent infections are among other possible reasons for inexplicable weight loss.

Asking for Medical Guidance:

People who lose weight for no apparent reason should get medical help right away. To identify the reason for the weight loss and, if necessary, start the appropriate therapy, a comprehensive examination, a review of the patient's medical history, and diagnostic testing can be required.

In conclusion, people should seek medical treatment if they have unexplained weight loss, particularly if it isn't brought on by a change in lifestyle. When it comes to possible health problems, such as the potential for cancer, early identification and management may be crucial.

Tiredness

Excessive and unexplained weariness that does not go away even after getting enough sleep may be a serious symptom of underlying health issues and may even be linked to some malignancies. This kind of fatigue, often known as cancer-related fatigue, is more than just the normal weariness that comes with daily living.

Features of Fatigue Associated with Cancer:

Extended and Unwavering:
One of the hallmarks of cancer-related tiredness is a chronic, unwavering feeling of weariness that lasts for a long time. This kind of exhaustion doesn't get better with more rest or sleep, unlike normal fatigue.

Not in Line with Activity Level:
Cancer-related fatigue sufferers may discover that their degree of exhaustion is not commensurate with their degree of physical or mental exertion. A severe feeling of exhaustion may arise from very little effort.

Not Reduced by Getting Sleep:
Cancer-related fatigue often lasts, and people may wake up feeling just as exhausted as when they went to bed, in contrast to the ordinary weariness that

may be relieved by getting a full night's sleep.

Interference with Day-to-Day Operations:

The weariness brought on by cancer might seriously impair one's capacity to carry out regular duties and activities. It's not just your average weariness that may be eased by brief pauses or rest.

Effect on Emotions:

Additionally, this kind of exhaustion may have emotional effects, making one feel irritable, moody, and less able to handle stress.

Possible Reasons:

Treatment for Cancer:
The adverse effects of cancer therapies including chemotherapy, radiation therapy, or immunotherapy are often

linked to weariness connected to cancer. Excessive fatigue may be attributed to the effects of these therapies on healthy cells as well as the body's reaction to them.

Cancer Per Se:

Fatigue-causing chemicals may be produced and metabolic alterations can occur when cancer is present in the body. Additionally, weariness may arise as a result of the body's immunological reaction to cancer.

Ahememia

Anemia, a disorder marked by a reduction in red blood cells, may be brought on by some malignancies. This disease impairs the amount of oxygen delivered to tissues and increases weariness.

Getting Medical Help:

It is important to take persistent and unexplained weariness seriously, particularly if it is severe. Seeking advice from a medical expert is essential for a thorough assessment. To ascertain the underlying reason, whether it is associated with cancer or another medical disease, diagnostic testing can be required. A better quality of life and a more successful treatment plan may result from early root cause diagnosis and management. It is advised that people who feel unusually tired speak honestly with their healthcare professionals so that a complete evaluation and suitable intervention may be made.

ALTERATIONS IN THE SKIN

Skin changes may be important markers of skin cancer, especially when it comes to changes in the color, size, or form of moles or the emergence of new skin lesions. Furthermore, jaundice—which is defined as a yellowing of the skin and eyes—may indicate the existence of certain kinds of pancreatic or liver tumors.

Modifications to Skin Lesions and Moles:

Color Shifts:

Attention should be paid to any discernible changes in the color of preexisting moles or the emergence of new ones. Uneven coloration, darkening, or lightening might be signs of aberrant cell development linked to skin cancer.

Size Variations:
It's crucial to keep an eye on mole size. Prompt expansion or a notable enlargement may be suggestive of cancerous alterations. A medical practitioner should check any mole that is bigger than the eraser of a pencil (6 mm or 1/4 inch).

Shape Shifts:
Concerns may arise from modifications to a mole's form, such as uneven borders or an uneven look. When determining whether or not a mole is normal, symmetry is crucial.

Crying or bruising:
Any moles that develop tenderness, itching, or bleeding without any obvious reason should be looked at right once. These symptoms need a dermatologist's evaluation since they could indicate aberrant cell activity.

YELLOWING OF THE SKIN WITH JAUNDICE:

***Discoloration of the Skin*:**
Increased amounts of the yellow pigment bilirubin cause jaundice, which appears as a yellow coloring of the skin and eyes. This may be a sign of problems with the liver or pancreas, including certain types of cancer that damage these organs.

Benign tumors of the pancreas or liver: Cancers of the liver or pancreas may block the bile ducts, which causes bilirubin to build up in the blood. The skin and eyes may get yellow as a consequence.

Associated Symptoms:
Other symptoms include pale stools, dark urine, stomach discomfort, and unexplained weight loss might coexist

with jaundice. All of these symptoms together call for a thorough medical assessment.

The Value of Quick Evaluation

Any significant changes to the skin, particularly those about moles and the onset of jaundice, should cause people to seek medical help right away. For skin cancer or tumors affecting the liver and pancreas to be effectively managed, early identification and action are essential.

When combined with expert dermatological assessments, regular skin self-examinations help to quickly identify any problems and may greatly enhance results. People who see any unusual changes in their skin or who are having symptoms related to jaundice should speak with medical specialists for a comprehensive evaluation and the proper course of treatment.

Continued Pain

Sustained pain that doesn't go away or doesn't go away with time might be a serious symptom of underlying medical conditions, such as malignancies of different kinds. Notably, persistent back or stomach discomfort may be a sign of some malignancies, including ovarian, colorectal, or pancreatic cancer.

Consistency in Pain Features:

Time and Reliability:

The hallmark of persistent pain is its protracted presence, which lasts longer than the typical time needed to heal after an accident or illness. Its recurrence or continuous nature raises questions about potential underlying medical issues.

Not connected to injury:
Persistent pain is not associated with a particular trauma or physical damage, in contrast to pain that has just arisen from an injury. It often has no obvious external source and may have an internal genesis.

Not Reduced by Silence:
Conventional pain management techniques like rest may not be effective in treating persistent pain. The soreness does not go away even after getting enough rest, which highlights the need to be checked out by a doctor.

RELATIONSHIP TO PARTICULAR CANCERS:

Cancer of the Pancreas:
Pancreatic cancer has been linked to persistent abdominal discomfort, especially in the upper abdomen or the

area around the back. Deep, enduring pain that often radiates to the back is possible with this kind of pain.

Hepatocellular Cancer:

Constant stomach pain or discomfort may be an indication of colorectal cancer, particularly if it is accompanied by chronic constipation or diarrhea. In the abdominal area, pain may be either localized or widespread.

Breast Cancer:

Persistent pelvic or abdominal discomfort is a possible side effect of ovarian cancer. People should pay attention to any inexplicable discomfort since it might be ill-defined and hard to pinpoint a particular reason for it.

The Value of Quick Evaluation

Early Recognition and Intervention:

For early diagnosis and management, timely identification of chronic pain is essential. Early cancer detection often improves the prognosis after therapy.

All-encompassing Medical Evaluation: People who are in pain all the time, particularly in the back or abdomen, should have a full medical evaluation. To find the underlying reason, this may include physical exams, imaging scans, and other diagnostic procedures.

Discard Other Circumstances:
It's crucial to remember that chronic pain may also be caused by non-cancerous illnesses, even though it may be linked to cancer. A comprehensive medical assessment aids in eliminating potential reasons and directs the right course of action.

Honest Communication with Medical Professionals:

People should be honest with their healthcare professionals about the kind, intensity, and features of their pain. To make an appropriate diagnosis and create a successful treatment strategy, this information is essential.

In conclusion, chronic pain that is not associated with a recognized injury and does not go away with time has to be carefully considered. Seeking quick medical treatment enables a thorough assessment, guaranteeing that any underlying health problems—including possible cancers—are found and treated as soon as possible.

Modifications to Bladder or Bowel Habits

Modifications in bowel or bladder habits may be significant markers of underlying health problems and, in some instances, may be linked to different forms of cancer. Notably, blood in the stool and ongoing diarrhea or constipation may be indicators of colorectal cancer. On the other hand, alterations in urine patterns may indicate malignancies of the bladder, prostate, or other organs.

alterations in bowel habits

Constant Diarrhea or Constipation:

Consistently experiencing constipation or diarrhea might be a sign of colorectal cancer, since they are evident and persistent changes in bowel patterns. These alterations are often long-lasting and difficult to attribute to transient diseases or dietary variables.
Stool Containing Blood:

Whether it is evident or picked up by stool testing, the presence of blood in the stool is a worrying indication. One possible reason for this might be colorectal cancer, and it could signal bleeding in the digestive system. Blood in the stool may also be caused by other illnesses including inflammatory bowel disease or hemorrhoids.

MODIFICATIONS TO URINARY HABITS:

BREAST CANCER:

Urination patterns may alter as a result of prostate cancer. Increased frequency of urination, trouble initiating or halting the flow, a feeble urine stream, or the impression that the bladder is not completely emptying are possible symptoms.

Colorectal Cancer:

Urinary abnormalities, such as hematuria—the presence of blood in the urine—may be a sign of bladder cancer. Urine with hematuria may look red, pink, or brownish. It's also possible to notice painful urination or frequent urine.

Different Cancers

Variations in the way one urinates may indicate the presence of further pelvic malignancies. For instance, bladder function abnormalities brought on by ovarian or uterine malignancies in women may result in increased urgency or frequency.

The Significance of Medical Assessment

Prompt Diagnosis:

Timely diagnosis depends on identifying and treating changes in bowel or bladder habits. Treatment results may be greatly impacted by early identification of tumors such as bladder, prostate, colorectal, or other cancers.

Exams for diagnosis:

To determine the underlying reason for changes in bowel or bladder habits, healthcare practitioners may offer a variety of diagnostic testing, such as imaging investigations, colonoscopies, or prostate-specific antigen (PSA) tests. Consultation with Medical Specialists:

People who notice consistent changes in their bladder or bowel habits should speak with medical specialists. The diagnosis approach is guided by open communication on the symptoms, duration, and any related circumstances.

Hazard Elements and Screening:

Early identification and prevention of some cancers depend on individuals being aware of their risk factors and taking part in suitable screening programs, such as prostate or colorectal cancer screenings.

In conclusion, it is important to pay attention to any changes in bowel or bladder habits since they may indicate malignancies or other underlying health problems. Obtaining early medical attention, talking with healthcare professionals about symptoms, and doing suggested testing may all help with early discovery and successful treatment.
Having Trouble Swallowing

Swallowing difficulties, or dysphagia as it is known in medicine, maybe a worrisome sign of several illnesses, including several malignancies of the stomach, throat, or esophagus.

Features of Troubles with Swallowing:

Perception of Damage:

People who have dysphagia may feel as if something is becoming caught in their chest or throat, giving them the impression of blockage.
Agony or Unease:

In addition to difficulty swallowing, soreness or discomfort in the chest, throat, or behind the breastbone may be experienced during the swallowing process.

Repetitions:

Some people who have dysphagia may cough up food particles or liquids, which may cause them to feel as if they are choking.

Dietary Loss:

If it prevents a person from eating normally, persistent trouble swallowing may lead to inadvertent weight loss. Connection to Cancers:

GASTRIC CANCER:

Swallowing difficulties are often a sign of esophageal cancer. Esophageal tumors may constrict the path, which makes it difficult for liquids and food to flow through.

PHARYNGEAL (THROAT) CANCER:

Swallowing difficulties may result from pharyngeal or throat cancers. The swallowing reflex may not function normally if there are tumors in this area.
Gastric Cancer:

Swallowing difficulties may sometimes be a sign of stomach cancer. Food transit may be hampered by tumors that affect the upper or lower portions of the stomach or esophagus.
The Value of Quick Evaluation

Fundamental Reasons:

Swallowing difficulties may arise from several reasons, not only cancer. To determine the underlying cause of this symptom, a comprehensive medical assessment is needed.

EXAMS FOR DIAGNOSIS:

Medical professionals may suggest procedures like barium swallow studies, endoscopies, or imaging scans to evaluate the anatomy and physiology of the esophagus and its environs.
Early Recognition and Intervention:

It is essential to discover malignancies early if swallowing difficulties are present to start treatment on time. Early intervention may improve the quality of life and treatment results.
Working together with medical professionals:

Patients who are having trouble swallowing should be transparent with their medical professionals, giving them as much information as possible regarding the kind and severity of their symptoms. This cooperation aids in directing the process of diagnosis and ensuing treatment planning.

NUTRITIONAL ASSISTANCE:

Healthcare professionals may suggest nutritional assistance or dietary changes to guarantee enough calorie and nutrient intake if difficulties swallowing make it difficult to maintain proper nutrition.

In conclusion, dysphagia, or trouble swallowing, is a symptom that should not be disregarded, particularly if it persists. It might be linked to several illnesses, such as stomach, throat, or esophageal malignancies. Finding the underlying reason and putting successful measures in place requires seeking prompt medical attention, getting the right diagnostic testing, and working with healthcare providers.

CHRONIC COUGH OR HOARSE VOICE

A chronic cough or hoarseness that does not go away with traditional treatment might be a good marker of other possible health problems, most notably lung or throat cancer.

Features of a Prolonged Cough or Hoarse Voice:

Length:

Long-lasting hoarseness or cough, usually lasting more than three weeks, is regarded as chronic and should be treated.

Strength:

The severity of the hoarseness or cough, particularly if it becomes worse over time, might make you worry about an underlying medical problem.

Not receptive to corrections:

A chronic cough or hoarseness that does not go away with rest, fluids, or over-the-counter drugs may be a sign of something more serious.
Connection to Cancers:

CHEST CANCER:

Lung cancer early symptoms may include a chronic cough. Lung tumors may irritate the airways, which can result in persistent coughing. There may also be other respiratory symptoms like chest discomfort or dyspnea.

Laryngeal Cancer of the Throat:

Vocal abnormalities, such as hoarseness, may be linked to laryngeal or throat cancer. Vocal cord tumors may be the cause of chronic hoarseness.
The Value of Quick Evaluation

Exams for diagnosis:

People who have a chronic cough or hoarse voice need to have a full medical examination. It could be advised to undertake diagnostic procedures like imaging studies or endoscopic exams to evaluate the anatomy of the throat and lungs.

Early Recognition and Intervention:

For lung or throat cancer to be treated promptly, early diagnosis is essential. Early-stage cancers often respond better to therapy and provide more alternatives. Hazard Elements and Screening:

It is crucial to comprehend one's unique risk factors for lung and throat cancers, such as the history of cancer, cigarette smoking, and exposure to environmental contaminants. Healthcare professionals may suggest suitable tests based on risk factors.
Working together with medical professionals:

It's critical to be open and honest with medical professionals about the length, severity, and accompanying symptoms of a chronic cough or hoarseness. This data aids in directing the process of diagnosis and ensuing therapy planning.

In conclusion, a chronic cough or hoarseness that doesn't go away over time might be a sign of more serious health issues, such as lung or throat cancer. Getting medical help as soon as possible, following approved diagnostic procedures, and working with medical experts are all crucial to determining the underlying reason and carrying out the right treatments.